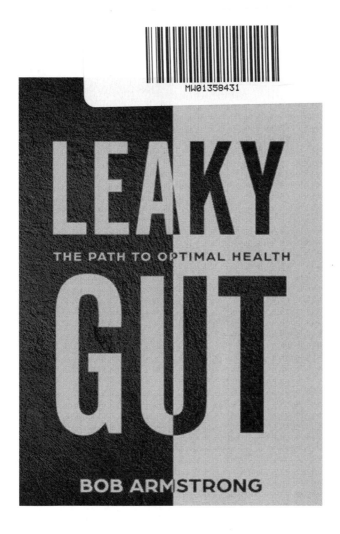

Leaky Gut
The Path to Optimal Health
Bob Armstrong

Copyright Bob Armstrong- First Edition © 2018

Cover design, texts and illustrations by Bob Armstrong used under license or are in the public domain. All rights reserved under US, International and Pan American Copyright Conventions. No portion of this book may be reproduced or transmitted in any form without the expressed written permission of the author or publisher.

ISBN: 9781977075499

Disclaimer: Always use caution when beginning a new nutrition or health regimen program. We recognize that not all protocols are suitable for everyone. Please check with your doctor if you have questions. We will not be responsible or liable for any injury sustained as a result of using any program presented and/or discussions on our blog, website, via email communications, books or in video format.

Leaky Gut...The Path To Optimal Health

Preface

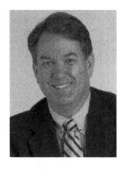

Welcome dear friend and thank you for your interest in this topic and for your purchase of this book. I hope that as you are suffering with this "leaky gut" condition that will find this information helpful. We have found that our gut is the gateway to health, and it houses 80% of your immune system, and you can't have a healthy immune system without a healthy gut. This book contains proven strategies on how to improve your gut health, so you can live a happy, healthy and rewarding life. Let's delve more into it shall we?

To begin, I have been interested in health and nutrition all of my life. I've been working as an integrative and holistic nutrition researcher and clinician since 2011. In working with my son, Dr.

Bob Armstrong of New Life Integrative of CA during this period, I have seen some amazing positive changes in the lives of our patients.

I'd like to share some of the best of my experiences along with insights from other leaders in the field of integrative, holistic, and functional medicine. The healthcare field is constantly changing. Over the last few years I've devoted much of my time to helping a new generation of patients anxious to know of practical, real-world alternative and functional solutions to many of their health issues. I hope to share additional information on some of these conditions as I release them soon. My goal is to thoroughly research problematic health conditions and share alternative solutions in an "easy-to-understand" way. Please keep coming back. You make the experience so worthwhile and joyful for everyone. I long ago recognized that knowledge is power wherever we find it, and when properly applied. Your understanding is vital to your progress. Keep researching and learning. It'

Always wishing you the best in life and in health.

Bob Armstrong

Acknowledgements

This book is dedicated to all of those who have inspired me throughout my life and to those who have encouraged me to ask the question "why." Albert Einstein once said "The important thing is not to stop questioning. Curiosity has its own reason for existing." And Walt Disney shared that "We keep moving forward, opening new doors, and doing new things, because we're curious and curiosity keeps leading us down new paths. So keep curious and make learning fun and enjoyable on your journey.

To my wife Denise who has been my rock and eternal companion and who continues to inspire and support me in all that I do. Thank you sweetheart. I love you so much.

To my son, Dr. Bob who has not only taught and practiced the principles in this book with delicate care for each of his patients, but for his guiding hand in challenging me to be all that I can be. His encouragement and love have always been an important part of his coaching and practice mentorship and I have been blessed to be a part of it. Thank you Bob.

And a special thank you to YOU! You are the reason for this book. It's you who may be suffering from "leaky gut" and that alone, changes your life to an extent. May you continue to be a student of your health? Remember, you know your health better than anyone else, including your doctor. Seek out all the best information you can from every good source that you can find; that you may create, for yourself, an optimal health lifestyle that not only adds years to your life, but gives life to your years. To yours in health always...thank you. Bob.

Table of Contents

Introduction 7

Chapter 1 - What is Leaky Gut?..11

Chapter 2 – Leaky Gut and Autoimmune Disorders..............22

Chapter 3 - Signs and Symptoms of Leaky Gut?...................30

Chapter 4 - Your Digestive Tract-What You Need to Know...33

Chapter 5 - Foods Linked to Leaky Gut..................................38

Chapter 6 - Probiotics Vs Prebiotics 44

Chapter 7 - Recovering from Leaky Gut...............................469

Chapter 8 - Herbs and Supplements That Can Help 89

Conclusion..117

Resources 1192

Please check out our other
Optimal Health Series
books as they become available.
Thank you!

Introduction

If you've been experiencing digestive issues recently, you could have leaky gut syndrome. If you have experienced an autoimmune condition such as lupus, rheumatoid arthritis, psoriatic arthritis or an irritable bowel syndrome, you might want to take a closer look at your gut, often called your "second brain."

Leaky gut is just now starting to come onto the radar for doctors as more and more of their patients are developing gastrointestinal and other disorders with no previous history or genetic predisposition. In this book, you will learn what leaky gut is, its potential causes, and proposed treatments that might be able to not only relieve your symptoms, but make leaky gut a thing of the past for you.

Let's dive in and get started with a definition of what leaky gut is first shall we?

Chapter 1 - What is Leaky Gut?

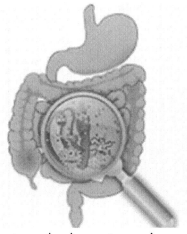

Leaky gut, or leaky gut syndrome, is not actually an agreed-upon medical condition. The medical term for it is *intestinal permeability*. When something is impermeable, it does not allow liquid to pass through, such as water. If something is permeable, it allows liquid to pass through, or leak.

Complementary and alternative medicine (CAM) practitioners have developed the theory that a leaky gut, that is, one which is overly permeable, releases various toxins, microbes, and even undigested food particles and other potentially harmful substances into the body, creating an inflammation response and sending white blood cells to fight the intruders in the blood system, leading to illness. They have speculated that a leaky gut might be connected with a range of health issues too, including:

- Acne
- Anxiety
- Arthritis
- Autism
- Autoimmune disorders
- Bloating
- Cancer
- Cardiovascular disorders
- Celiac disease
- Constipation
- Crohn's disease
- Decreased immune function

- Depression
- Diabetes
- Diarrhea
- Eczema
- Gas
- Heartburn
- Hypothyroidism
- Intestinal pain
- Inflammatory bowel disease (IBD)
- Irritable bowel syndrome (IBS)
- Joint pain
- Metabolic syndrome
- Mood swings
- Muscle pain
- Osteoporosis
- Psoriasis
- Psoriatic arthritis and more

If we look at this list, some of these are symptoms of a leaky gut. We might thing some of the conditions are completely logical, such as leaky gut being connected with gastrointestinal issues such as:

- Bloating
- Celiac disease
- Constipation
- Crohn's disease
- Gas
- Heartburn
- Intestinal pain
- Inflammatory bowel disease (IBD) and
- Irritable bowel syndrome (IBS)

We can also understand that what we eat and how it is digested is important in relation to diabetes and metabolic syndrome. For those of you who are not familiar with metabolic syndrome, it is five related conditions that are thought to be a precursor of insulin resistance, which is thought to be a sign of diabetes. The 5 conditions that could indicate you have metabolic syndrome are:

1. High blood pressure
2. High cholesterol
3. High triglycerides (a certain type of cholesterol)
4. High blood sugar
5. Waist roundness, that is, a 'spare tire' around your middle, which can often be a sign of being overweight, another common symptom amongst those with metabolic syndrome.

A diagnosis of metabolic syndrome is usually made on the basis of 3 of these factors being present. As the name suggests, something is going on with the metabolism. This starts to cause poor health, and could potentially be the way the body is using, or losing, the nutrients it is taking in, which could be the result of a leaky gut.

But is it really possible for our digestive tract to be connected to autism? New research has shown that autism might be connected to autoimmune issues and chemical imbalances that result, as well as the genetic components of autism that have already been researched.

Even though there is no specific diagnosis of leaky gut, doctors do know that certain things can affect the permeability of the intestines and throw the microbiome, that is, gut flora, out of balance. These include:

- Overuse of antibiotics
- Using non-steroidal anti-inflammatory drugs (NSAIDs), such as aspirin and ibuprofen
- Taking Proton-pump inhibitors (PPIs), which reduce gastric acid production
- A poor diet that damages the microbiome
- A poor diet that lacks the nutrients needed to maintain a healthy microbiome
- Too much sugar

- Genetically modified foods (GMOs)
- Stress
- Tap water
- Mercury, such as in canned fish
- BPA, such as in plastic bottles we drink from
- Pesticides
- Yeast infections (Candida)

Food-borne illnesses can also trigger leaky gut, including:

Norovirus, a highly contagious stomach bug passed from person to person through bodily fluids such as saliva, vomit, diarrhea, and poor hand washing practices. It is known as the curse of cruise ships because of frequent outbreaks and the ease of transmission in confined spaces.

Salmonella, which comes from contaminated or undercooked foods, such as chicken and eggs, and from certain pets, including turtles, birds, and handling pet foods and then not washing your hands carefully afterwards.

Giardiasis, from the parasite Giardia, the most common stomach parasite in the US. It comes from water contaminated with fecal matter.

There are many more food-borne illness such as E. Coli, listeria, cyclospora, shigella that can have a significant impact on your gut. Some of these will resolve on their own. In other cases, they may require antibiotics. In still other cases, doctors will give a broad spectrum antibiotic to cover all contingencies. The trouble with this is that antibiotics of any kind will change the gut flora, killing helpful bacteria as well as harmful ones.

Doctors prescribing antibiotics "just in case," or because pressured to do so by patients who insist on getting a pill of some sort when they go to the doctor, has given rise to antibiotic-resistant 'super bugs' and in some cases, serious damage to the microbiome. One recent study has shown that one course of antibiotics can kill off so many bacteria that the flora still haven't recovered two years later.

One of the most serious forms of damage is Clostridium difficile (C. difficile, or C. diff) colitis, which is an overgrowth of C diff bacteria in your gut. This bacteria releases toxins that attack the lining of the intestines. Though relatively rare compared to other intestinal bacteria, C. diff is one of the most important causes of infectious diarrhea in the US.

The most common symptoms are severe abdominal pain and watery diarrhea, sometimes with blood and pus in it, up to 15 times a day. Such extreme loss of bodily fluids can lead to dehydration and death. Another potentially fatal symptom of C diff is if the bacteria forms an actual hole in the intestine.

At this point, C diff can really only be treated via fecal transplant. That is, the feces from a healthy person is inserted into the colon of a person with C diff in the hope of rebalancing the gut flora. However, getting enough healthy feces for transplantation has proven to be a problem, demonstrating just how many American digestive systems are in poor condition.

Studies are bringing us closer to an understanding of just how sophisticated our gut is. For example, did you know that 90% of our digestion takes place in our small intestine, NOT in our stomach? Therefore, a leaky gut can have serious health implications if left untreated. It is often said that our stomachs are our "second brain". Here's a fascinating BBC broadcast that shows how our food travels through the stomach and

through the intestine as recorded with a small lighted-camera pill.
https://www.youtube.com/watch?v=5ufESc1bK78

Now that we know what leaky gut is, what illnesses it is connected to, and a number of the potential causes of leaky gut syndrome, let's look at how it is connected to autoimmune disorders.

Chapter 2 – Leaky Gut and Autoimmune Disorders

CAM practitioners are pretty sure that leaky gut syndrome exists. What they don't know is what affect that permeability has on one's overall health. Gastrointestinal disorders can produce a wide range of symptoms, many of which seem unrelated to the digestive system:

We would all love to be able to go to the doctor, get a definitive diagnosis, and be given a pill and told exactly what to do to cure ourselves. In the case of leaky gut, it is just one sign of many potential underlying medical disorders. On the other hand, it might be a chicken-and-egg issue. Is the leaky gut a result of the disease? Or the disease the cause of the leaky gut?

While some of this might sound like weird science, until more research is done, CAM practitioners and mainstream doctors interested in the theory, and in nutrition and/or autoimmune disorders, have to work with patients to track their symptoms and note their diet, lifestyle and habits. In this way they can try to narrow down what might be causing the leaky gut and any other illness they might be suffering from.

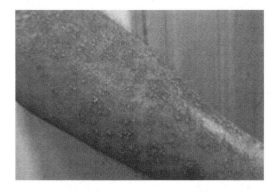

It is important to note that many of the illnesses on the list in the previous chapter that might be associated with leaky gut have an autoimmune component. That is, they involve inflammation, something irritating the body in some way, which will often cause the immune system to attack the body it is supposed to be protecting. The theory is that the substances leaking from the gut are perceived as threats by the immune system, which goes into full defense mode due to the leakage.

According to the American Autoimmune Related Diseases Association, approximately 50 million Americans have some form of autoimmune disorder. More than 80 different conditions come under this umbrella. They include:

- Graves' disease (fast thyroid)
- Hashimoto's disease (slow thyroid)
- Rheumatoid arthritis (RA)
- Systemic lupus erythematosus (SLE, or lupus)
- Multiple sclerosis (MS) and many more

It is important to note that 90% of RA and SLE cases are in women. In terms of MS, women are 3 times more likely to contract it than men. Is there a hormonal component? Or are women's diets literally diets, unnatural ways of eating that rely on artificial sweeteners and other chemicals in an effort to control or lose weight, which are really damaging their gut and metabolism?

Some of these autoimmune disorders have symptoms in common. While these diseases are generally viewed as separate conditions, they share common causes. One of the main ones is the immune system having a hard time distinguishing friend from foe, resulting in the body starting to attack itself.

As the body's primary defense against disease and infection, the immune system is connected to all other biological systems. As a result, the immune system being turned 'on' and staying on can cause damage throughout the body, resulting in what is termed chronic systemic inflammation (CSI). CSI confuses and damages the immune system even more, leading to even greater dysfunction.

Therefore, rather than try to treat specific conditions one at a time, a holistic approach that gets to the bottom of the inflammation and autoimmune response could clear up multiple conditions. For example, men with prostate disorders also tend to have coronary heart disease and arthritis. Is it possible that what is causing the hardening of the arteries (arteriosclerosis) is related to the arthritis and prostate issues? Since we know arteriosclerosis is triggered by inflammation, as is arthritis, it's perfectly possible it could be related to prostate problems as well.

Since we are what we eat, our diet is a key factor in our overall health. If we have a leaky gut, however, we are failing to get the nutrients we need and the food and substances we are taking into our body through the food. The water and food we consume then can literally be poisoning us and causing our own body to attack these 'invaders', doing even more damage.

While the causes of autoimmune diseases are not fully known, many triggers have been identified, including:

- microorganisms, such as bacteria or viruses
- environmental factors such as pollution
- medications and over-the-counter pain relievers
- chemical irritants
- intestinal permeability
- food sensitivities

- unhealthy foreign bodies that look similar to healthy cells, which confuse the immune system and cause both to be attacked
- genetic predisposition- a family history of arthritis or heart disease, for example, seems to make a person more prone to developing these illness themselves.

As we learn more about genetic components of disease, it can be easy for people to become discouraged and think that they are doomed. That there is nothing they can do to avoid becoming ill. But the truth is that making healthy choices can offset the genetic risks, making it less likely you will fall ill.

One of the best ways to prevent a disease is to know what causes it, and take action to counteract it. Even if you can't prevent the disease, knowing the signs and symptoms can help you spot the condition early so it doesn't progress into something serious that will be much harder, if not impossible, to treat later on.

Chapter 3 - Signs and Symptoms of Leaky Gut?

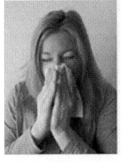

There are a number of signs and symptoms of a leaky gut. Many of them are linked to gastrointestinal issues, but some are more general overall health issues. They include:

- Digestive issues such as gas, bloating, diarrhea, constipation
- Irritable bowel syndrome (IBS)
- Depression
- Fatigue
- Fever
- General malaise (feeling ill)
- Seasonal allergies
- Asthma
- Muscle aches
- Inflammation such as redness, heat, pain, and swelling

- Hormonal imbalances such as pre-menstrual syndrome (PMS) or Polycystic Ovarian Syndrome (PCOS).
- Celiac disease
- Crohn's disease
- Diagnosed chronic fatigue syndrome (CFS)
- Diagnosed fibromyalgia
- Mood disorders such as depression and anxiety
- Attention Deficit-Hyperactivity Disorder (ADHD) or Attention Deficit Disorder (ADD)
- Skin issues such as acne, rosacea, eczema or psoriasis
- Diagnosis of candida overgrowth (yeast infection)
- Food allergies, sensitivities and intolerances, such as to gluten
- Diagnosis of an autoimmune disease such as:
- Rheumatoid arthritis
- Hashimoto's thyroiditis
- Lupus

- Psoriatic arthritis

It's important to not try to relieve one symptom at a time, but rather, look at the problem holistically. Let's take a quick look at what you need to know about your digestive tract so you can grasp the potential effects of a leaky gut.

Also, it is quite common with leaky gut present, to have several autoimmune conditions at one time. Many of the above autoimmune conditions show up together. It's not uncommon, for example, to have an irritable Bowel Syndrome, constant digestive issues, Celiac disease and Psoriasis condition, all showing up at the same time. Stress, poor dietary food selection, combined with a leaky gut condition can be just the combination to create havoc in your system.

Chapter 4 - Your Digestive Tract-What You Need to Know

You probably take your digestive tract for granted, but it is an amazingly complex system with varied functions that extends from your mouth all the way to your anus.

You start digesting the moment you put food into your mouth. Your teeth and saliva start breaking down the food so it can travel down the esophagus to the stomach. Think of your digestive system as a finely-tuned conveyor belt, with the muscles within your stomach and intestines moving the food along to each important stage of digestion. This movement is called motility.

In the stomach are acids that digest the food even further so your small intestine will be able to remove the nutrients from the food and send them out to the rest of the body. The large intestine, or color, will help get rid of the rest as waste products, which are removed through the process of urination (elimination) and excretion (stool, feces, excrement).

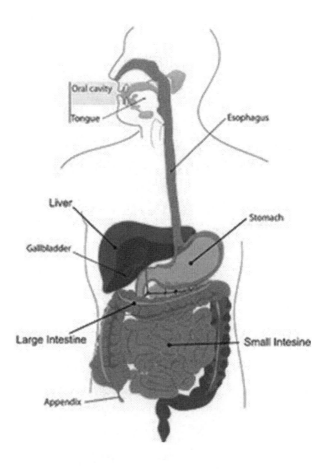

Digestive juices contain enzymes that break food down into different nutrients. The small intestine is responsible for 90% of your digestion, so a leaky gut can be a disaster for the body. In addition to releasing toxic substances, it will fail to absorb nutrients. Without essential nutrients, you will become ill.

The walls of the small intestine allow the nutrients into the bloodstream, which delivers them to the rest of the body. Therefore, we know the small intestine is permeable. However, if it is too permeable, your gut can leak into the body cavity. Hormone and nerve regulators control the digestive process, for example, signaling when you feel full, and when to release insulin.

Your food traveling from your mouth to your anus is a long journey of nearly 70 yards that involves a range of enzymes and digestive juices and about 1,000 different bacteria, many of them helpful, some of them harmful if they get out of control, such as C diff.

On such a long and complicated journey, a lot can go wrong. Therefore, taking a closer look at what you put in your mouth is the best way to decrease the risk of leaky gut and increase your digestive health. In the next chapter, we'll look at foods that doctors believe contribute to leaky gut syndrome.

Chapter 5 - Foods Linked to Leaky Gut

There are a number of foods and other things we consume that are related to leaky gut.

- Cow's milk and products made from it
- Whole grain wheat
- Glutens
- Genetically Modified and Hybrid Foods
- Tap water with chlorine and/or fluoride
- Sugar, and items that are perceived as sugar by the body
- Artificial sweeteners
- Artificial colorings
- Salt
- Preservatives
- Too much yeast in the diet
- Alcoholic beverages

Due to the food industry in the US and developed nations, many of these items are in the foods we eat without us even realizing them. Labels can be confusing and the manufacturers know all the loopholes. Cow's milk is used for taste and moisture. It's also powdered and therefore highly concentrated, and is used in all sorts of foods as a thickener.

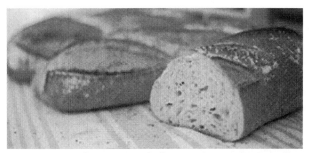

So too is wheat, and the protein from the wheat, gluten. If you've ever tried to eat low-carb, you will know how hard it can be because wheat and carbs, like sugar, are everywhere. Gluten is often labeled as food starch or modified food starch.

GMO and other engineered foods are bred to be sturdier, yield more, and be insect-resistant. This undoubtedly affects their make-up and digestibility. So to do the pesticides that are used on them and the water that helps grow them.

Some nutritionist's term processed cane sugar, as 'white death' because of its damaging effects on the body. This has led people to turn to what they think are healthier alternatives, such as honey, agave nectar and brown rice syrup. They are mistaken. The body still treats them as sugar. And brown rice syrup is typically heavily contaminated with arsenic, due to the water in the rice paddies where the rice grows, being contaminated.

Artificial sweeteners are all man-made using chemicals. Stevia is a natural sweetener that is said to be safe and is far sweeter than sugar. In its natural form, it looks, smells and tastes like alfalfa. Unfortunately, this means it's not that versatile, so it gets heavily processed to make it look like white sugar. Stevia still appears to be the best sweetener choice today for those suffering with leaky gut.

Artificial coloring is yet another source of chemicals in the diet. Just think of the colors of Jell-O, Fruit Loops cereal, or

Kool-Aid and you will get an idea of just how full of chemicals convenience foods can be, and what America is feeding our younger generation, or even eating themselves.

Salt makes food taste better. It is also used as a cheap preservative, for example, in cold cuts, cheeses, and smoked products such as salmon, bacon and ham. Cold cuts also have other preservatives such as nitrates and nitrites. Aim for low sodium foods. Though our bodies need sodium to function properly, an overabundance of salt can be detrimental.

Alcoholic beverages are created via yeast turning sugar into alcohol. Both the sugar and yeast have been linked to leaky gut. Candida control may be vital to getting your gut under control. It's estimated that 70-80% of Americans have candida in some form, but it's not all bad. A very small amount of candida lives in your mouth and intestines and helps out with digestion and nutrient absorption.

But, "Invasive candidiasis" is a fungal infection that can occur when Candida yeasts enter the bloodstream. These can have detrimental effects. For example, when candida is overproduced, it can break down the walls of the intestine and penetrate the bloodstream — releasing toxic by-products into your body and causing leaky gut and candidiasis (candida infection). This can lead to many different health problems, from digestive issues to autoimmune conditions.

Now that you know several of the most harmful foods in relation to leaky gut, what can be done to improve your digestion? Let's look at probiotics in the next chapter.

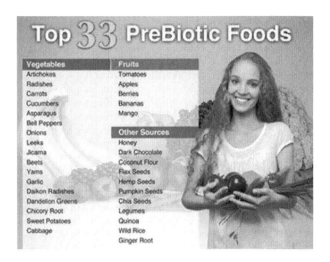

Chapter 6 - Probiotics Vs. Prebiotics

In recent years, more and more people have started to understand the importance of probiotics for the digestion. Bacteria in the digestive tract help digest the food and keep the intestine healthy. These bacteria are commonly referred to as gut flora.

However, gut flora can be disrupted and even killed off due to certain food and medications, in particular, antibiotics. Antibiotics have been overprescribed in recent years, with increasingly serious consequences.

Probiotics can help restore the balance and prebiotics are what they live on. Increasing attention is now being paid to the best prebiotics to help the probiotics do their work.

Prebiotics

Prebiotics should be part of a balanced diet. However, a lot of people have adopted a low-carb diet, or a gluten-free one, thus eliminating one of the main sources of prebiotics, whole grain wheat. But there are other options that are not grain-based, including:

- Artichokes
- Asparagus
- Bananas
- Chicory

- Garlic
- Leeks
- Onion
- Potatoes
- Soy beans

Probiotics

Lactobacillus acidophilus and Bifid bacterium lactis are recommended for maintaining gut flora. They can be found in Greek-style yogurt, and in kefir, a fermented dairy drink. Just watch out for a lot of added sugar in these products.

Some people buy expensive probiotics in the refrigerator section of a good health food store, but there's really no need to when yogurt is so cheap.

Avoiding antibiotics is another aspect to the importance of the probiotics as an essential part of healthy gut flora.

The purpose of probiotics, whether in food or in supplement form, is to help improve the amount of beneficial bacteria in your gut. If you eat processed foods or foods with added sugars for example, they will do the opposite of what you want: they will nourish the potentially pathogenic bacteria in your gut. The bad guys love simple sugars.

On the other hand, pathogenic bacteria can't thrive on and derive the energy they need for growth from healthy fats, proteins, complex carbohydrates, and fiber-containing foods, (in other words a healthy diet). When you focus on eating *real food* that isn't processed or doesn't contain added sugars, you're supporting the growth of your good, beneficial bacteria.

So, what can you do to recover from leaky gut syndrome? Let's look at some all-natural ways in the next chapter.

Chapter 7 - Recovering from Leaky Gut

So is Leaky Gut repairable? Absolutely. The first step is to eliminate your triggers, such as poor dietary choices and stress. Other triggers can include painkillers like ibuprofen or aspirin (NSAIDS) and drinking too much alcohol. Once you've begun working on the elimination process, begin taking an L-Glutamine supplement. L-Glutamine is the fuel of the cell lining of the intestine and it helps regenerate your cells. It's good to know also, that intestinal tissue is one of the fastest healing tissues in the body. The key is to learn how to meet the unique needs of your body. Use a food journal to track those times when you feel bad, and see if you can spot a pattern. That will go a long way toward helping you reach a diagnosis and find a way to eliminate your condition. It can be a difficult learning experience, but one that's worth it to help you feel your best every day.

Here's are 5 steps that can help you recover from a leaky gut. They are:

1-RECOGNIZE the symptoms
2-REMOVE foods and factors that damage the gut
3-REPLACE the damaging foods with healing foods
4-REPAIR your leaky gut with specific herbs and supplements
5-REBALANCE your gut flora with prebiotics and probiotics and helpful enzymes

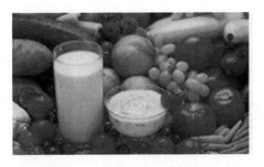

Recognize

Determine whether or not you have leaky gut. As of this point there are only a few test for Leaky Gut. The most common leaky gut test is called the "Lactulose/Mannitol. Test." 2) Then there's also a cool new technology in Cyrex Labs Array #2 "Intestinal Antigenic Permeability Screen." Both tests have their benefits but many doctors won't even look for it as an explanation.

Trust your knowledge of your own body. If you've been feeling drained, lacking in energy and generally feeling unwell, clearly something is going on. In which case, it's time to recognize there is something wrong with your health, and it's time to track what's going on, and make a change.

Once you've recognized that there is an issue, it's time to try to resolve it. The best place to start is to remove foods that might be causing your leaky gut issues. You might consider fasting for a day or 2 and then reintroducing these foods one at a time. Working with an allergy specialist can also help. So could a nutritionist and a CAM practitioner such as a DO or DC.

Different diets that could help with leaky gut

There are a number of eating lifestyles that might help with leaky gut.

Clean eating

Clean eating is latest buzz phrase among health-conscious consumers and emphasizes eating healthy, whole, unprocessed foods. It's like getting back to basics, eliminating all convenience foods and cooking from scratch. They will cook their food in such a way as to get maximum nutrition from it, such as making soups and stews and steaming the food lightly. Stove top cooking has proven to be a better choice than microwave use for stabilizing nutrients as well.

Raw diet

In a raw diet, as the name suggests, you don't cook your food in any way. Instead, you consume a lot of vegetables, fruits, seeds and nuts.

Organic diet

In some cases, people go organic, buying only products which are certified organic because they will not be exposed to pesticides, commercial fertilizer, and other chemicals that might get absorbed into the food and then into the body. Buying organic can be expensive, but shopping in warehouse clubs and growing your own food can help keep costs down. Higher quality, organically grown food is better absorbed in the body as well. An organic diet without the additives and pesticides is just better.

Gluten-free

Many people are going gluten-free. Gluten is a protein found in wheat, rye and barley. It is like the glue that holds the food together. The food industry uses gluten for texture and consistency or 'mouth feel' of food. You will often see it on labels as starch or modified food starch. Seek out gluten-free products where you can.

The Anti-inflammatory diet

Another promising way to deal with your leaky gut is to try an anti-inflammatory diet. This has been shown to be effective in relation to medical conditions that manifest with extreme inflammation, such as arthritis. If an anti-inflammatory diet can help arthritis pain, it could well be worth a try for your leaky gut.

There are two main principles to an anti-inflammatory diet. The first is to avoid foods believed to cause inflammation. The second is to add foods to your diet that are known to relieve inflammation. Swapping the good foods for the bad can keep you satisfied instead of miserable and deprived. They are tasty and could even help you lose weight.

Your food journal

Many people with health issues keep a journal of symptoms and actions, so they can see if what they are eating, for example, has any effect on the way they feel. A food journal is a great idea if you think you have a leaky gut. Eat as you normally would for your first couple of days. Then fast for a couple of days, such as doing a juice fast with carrot and other juices, or a soup fast with bone broth or other clear homemade soups. Then start your anti-inflammatory diet, making changes and jot down your results for each.

Here are 10 to avoid and 10 to try:

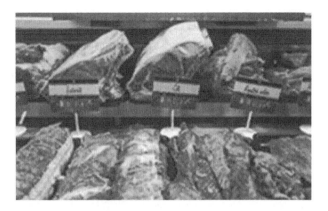

10 Foods to Avoid

1- Sugar and sugary foods like honey, agave and brown rice syrup, and fructose, such as high fructose corn syrup

2- Salt, commonly listed as sodium or nitrates on food labels

3- Standard Cooking Oils such as corn, safflower and vegetable oil

4- Red Meat such as beef and lamb, game meats like bison, boar and venison, and organ meats, such as heart, brains, kidneys and liver (all connected with gout, a very painful form of arthritis)

5- Processed Meats/Cold Cuts such as sliced roast beef or ham, because they are full of salt and chemical preservatives

6- Refined Carbohydrates such as cake, cookies and candies, white bread, white pasta

7- Full-fat Dairy Products such as milk, butter, cream, cottage cheese, yogurt and soft cheeses. Note that most cheese is very high in salt as well, which is used to preserve it.

8- Artificial Sweeteners and Flavorings, such as aspartame (NutraSweet, Equal), and Monosodium Glutamate (MSG)

9- Alcohol, due to the inflammatory effects on the body, plus chemicals such as sulfites that are used to preserve and stabilize wine

10- Trans fats, that are trans fatty acids.

There are two types of trans-fats found in foods: naturally-occurring and artificial trans-fats. Naturally-occurring trans-fats are produced in the gut of some animals and foods made from these animals, such as milk and meat products.

But the main source is man-made, that is created artificially through the process of adding hydrogen molecules to liquid vegetable oils in order to make them more solid.

Trans-fats are commonly labeled partially hydrogenated oils. They are added to convenience foods like cookies, crackers and other snacks to make them shelf-stable so they won't spoil. They also add texture and what is termed "mouth-feel" to these foods in order to make them tastier.

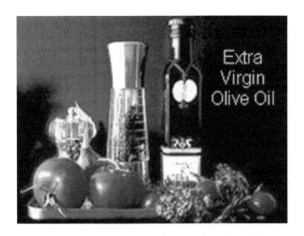

10 Foods to Add to Your Menus

1- Olive Oil (Extra virgin if you don't mind the stronger taste)-it is a fat so it should be used sparingly, but it has no cholesterol. Regular olive oil can be used as a substitute for most recipes calling for butter or margarine

2- Cherries, sweet, and tart (highly recommended if you have arthritis)

3- Walnuts and other tree nuts (if you are not allergic)

4- Bell peppers, such as green, red and yellow

5- Ginger, fresh root or dried-great in Indian and Chinese food

6- Turmeric, fresh root or dried- great in Indian food and rice dishes

7- Berries such as blueberries, raspberries and strawberries

8- Probiotics such as yogurt with live cultures and kefir, a cultured and fermented beverage made from dairy

9- Salmon and Other Fatty Fish with Omega-3 fatty acids

Salmon is just one fatty fish that is rich in Omega-3 fatty acids, which are said to be heart-healthy and reduce inflammation. Popular fish that are family- and budget friendly include:

•Alaskan Salmon, Wild, not farmed
•Arctic Char
•Atlantic Mackerel
•Bass
•Catfish
•Flounder
•Haddock
•Halibut
•Herring
•Pollock
•Red Snapper
•Sardines
•Sole
•Swordfish
•Trout

Some of these can have more than 1500 mg per 3 ounce serving. The daily allowance is 2,000 for ordinary people, up to 4,000 for athletes. Here's a handy chart of Omega-3 content in mg per 3 ounce serving:
http://www.seafoodhealthfacts.org/seafood-nutrition/healthcare-professionals/omega-3-content-frequently-consumed-seafood-products

Other sources like shark, king mackerel and tilefish are rich sources, but tend to be high in mercury and other toxins, so eat sparingly.

Fish can be expensive, so check your local warehouse club store. Steer clear of anything with a lot of breading on it or salty sauces.

Not real crazy about fish? Non-fishy sources of Omega-3s include:

•canola oil

- flaxseed-a tiny, crunchy, nutty seed that adds taste and texture to salads and baked goods
- flaxseed oil
- mustard seeds and greens, with the seeds used in Indian cooking and the greens boiled up like collard greens
- pumpkin seeds
- soybeans (tofu, edamame bean)
- soybean oil
- spinach
- walnuts
- wheat germ (found in whole grain wheat)

You can also get Omega-3 fatty acid supplements. The recommended daily allowance is 2000mg, so try to get it mainly from the food you eat. There's no need for mega doses. In fact, too much has been linked with heart health issues.

Fish oil supplements can also be expensive and not always very pure. Look for US or Canadian products. Krill oil and salmon oil should be very pure and safe and with the highest levels of Omega-3s.

10. Green leafy vegetables and cruciferous vegetables

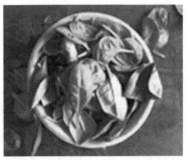

All vegetables are good for us because of the fiber and moisture helping us feel full, but there are a couple of classes that are most beneficial, green leafy vegetables and cruciferous vegetables.

Green leafy vegetables

There's a craze for kale these days as a green leafy food. It's being put into everything from soup to snacks. But there are lots of other options, some with an even better nutritional profile than kale. Add these to your menu too:

- Beet Greens
- Chicory
- Endive
- Iceberg lettuce
- Napa Cabbage
- Parsley
- Radicchio
- Romaine Lettuce
- Swiss Chard
- Spinach

Cruciferous vegetables

Cruciferous vegetables take their name from the cross shape they tend to grow in. Here are some tasty ones you will find easy to add to your meals. They are also quite filling and full of flavor, so they may help you lose weight.

- Arugula-this has a spicy, peppery taste and is great in salads

- Bok Choy (Chinese cabbage, great in stir fries)
- Broccoli
- Broccoli rabe
- Brussels sprouts
- Cabbage
- Cauliflower
- Collard greens
- Daikon (Japanese radish, nice with fish)
- Horseradish, such as in shrimp cocktail sauce
- Kale
- Mustard seeds, such as black mustard seeds (often used in Indian cooking)
- Mustard leaves
- Radish
- Rutabaga (Swedish turnip, or swede, orange in color)
- Turnips, root and greens
- Watercress-this has a peppery taste and is great in salads and with egg salad sandwiches

Vitamins and Minerals

Since leaky gut affects the absorption of nutrients from your food, it can start to lead to deficiencies, which can in turn worsen your leaky gut, creating a vicious cycle. When planning your meals, try to focus on natural sources of the following nutrients.

- Vitamin A
- Vitamin B, including B12
- Vitamin C
- Vitamin E
- Magnesium
- Iron
- Zinc

Here are a few suggestions regarding the main sources for each:

Vitamin A

Vitamin A is fat soluble, so it can be stored in the body. If you are looking for natural sources, think deep green, or orange foods.

- Butternut squash
- Beef liver
- Cantaloupe
- Carrots
- Kale
- Mangoes
- Pumpkins
- Spinach
- Sweet potatoes

Vitamin B, including B12

B vitamins are important because they are water-soluble, which means they can't be stored in the body. They are also important if you smoke cigarettes or are under a lot of stress, because these make you use up B vitamins even faster. B can also be tricky because they are an entire family of vitamins from B1 to 12. The most notable ones are

Vitamin B1   (thiamine)
Vitamin B3   (niacin)
Vitamin B5   (pantothenic acid)
Vitamin B6   (pyridoxine)
Vitamin B7   (biotin)
Vitamin B9   (folic acid)
Vitamin B12 (cobalamins)

B9

The most well-known is probably folic acid, since it is connected with healthy pregnancies. Main sources of B9 are:

- Asparagus
- Avocado
- Beans, such as black-eyed beans
- Broccoli
- Lentils
- Lettuce
- Mango
- Oranges
- Spinach

B12

B12 is not well-absorbed when a person suffers from leaky gut.

Mains sources of B12 include:
- Fortified Cereals (but watch out for too much sugar)
- Mackerel
- Milk
- Salmon
- Sardines
- Soy (tofu, edamame)
- Swiss cheese
- Yogurt

It is important to note that excessive amounts of B9 and B12 in pregnancy have recently been linked with a significantly greater risk of autism, so remember, supplement, but don't overdose
or treat vitamins as if they are a substitute for a healthy diet.

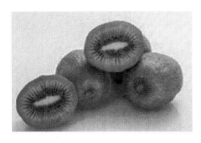

Vitamin C

Vitamin C is also water-soluble, so you need to replenish your supply every day. Fortunately, this is pretty easy to do, with a range of tasty foods. If you are not eating these foods daily, then supplementation is recommended. Here are a few natural sources:

- Bell peppers, yellow
- Berries, such as strawberries
- Broccoli
- Guava
- Kale
- Kiwi fruits
- Oranges (try to focus on the fruit, not a lot of juice)
- Papaya
- Peas
- Tomatoes

Vitamin E

Vitamin E maintains the walls of your cells and keeps skin healthy. It might contribute to maintaining the gut so it doesn't leak.

- Almonds
- Avocado
- Broccoli
- Kale
- Nuts like peanuts
- Olives
- Parsley
- Papaya
- Pumpkin seeds
- Spinach
- Swiss chard

Magnesium

Magnesium is an essential mineral used in many bodily function. Top sources include:

- Avocados
- Bananas
- Brown rice
- Dark chocolate
- Low-fat dairy
- Dried figs
- Mackerel
- Pollock
- Pumpkin seeds
- Soy beans
- Spinach

Iron

Iron is essential for healthy blood and circulation. Top sources to try include:

- Beans
- Beef or chicken liver
- Broccoli
- Clams
- Halibut
- Haddock
- Lentil

- Oysters
- Pumpkin seeds
- Spinach
- Salmon
- Sardines
- Spinach
- Tofu
- Tuna
- Turkey

Zinc

Zinc is required by many tissues and bodily functions. It also works in conjunction with magnesium to keep the brain sharp, which can help those with leaky gut who complain about a brain fog. Main sources include:

- Almonds
- Baked beans
- Beef
- Cashews
- Cheese, Swiss

- Chicken
- Chickpeas
- Crabmeat
- Flounder
- Kidney beans
- Oatmeal
- Peas
- Pork
- Pumpkin seeds
- Yogurt

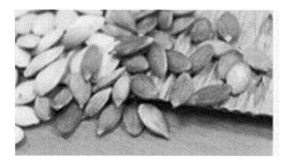

A good multivitamin can help cover anything missing from the food you eat, but again, don't overdo it, as too many vitamins and minerals can lead to overdose and other health issues. An age-related formula like Centrum Silver for seniors can also help keep you in balance. You can buy many types relatively inexpensively through a warehouse club.

Reducing stress

One other really key aspect to improving your digestive health is to reduce strategy in your life. There are a number of ways to relieve stress and improve your health, body, mind and spirit. Here are 15 top ones to try:

1- Set priorities. Focus on what's important and let go of the other stuff.

2- Identify tasks that you can share or delegate, then ask for help. Don't try to do everything yourself.

3- Get organized. Disorder can eat up time and make things tough to remember.

4- Don't try to multitask. There's no such things. It is just your brain switching back and forth between tasks. This leads to a lot of stress. Things take twice as long to do in the end compared to just doing one thing at a time from start to finish.

5- Set short-term goals you can reach. Then reward yourself when you meet them with something fun and relaxing.

6- Learn how to say no gracefully but firmly so you don't overextend yourself. Only agree to obligations that align with your priorities and inner truth.

7- Maintain a positive attitude. Choose to look for the good in others and yourself. Choose to make the best of any challenge you face rather than looking on the dark side.

8- Avoid perfectionism. Remember, things don't have to be perfect. Sometimes "good enough" is just fine.

9- Set aside some time, even 5 to 10 minutes, for yourself each day, to just sit and do nothing, or do something you love.

10-   Laugh more. Look for humor in your everyday life, or watch a funny movie.

11-   Listen to music. Choose tunes that relax or make you feel uplifted.

12-   Get things off your chest. Talk to a counselor or a friend.

13-   Get regular exercise. Find something you like doing that you can work into your schedule.

14-   Eat well. You can't put in your best performance if you're running on an empty fuel tank.

15-   Take a time-out for meditation, visualization, mindfulness, deep breathing, yoga, tai chi, and other stress-relief techniques.

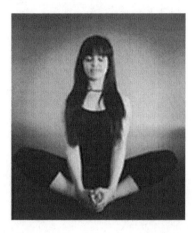

Meditation

Meditation is a practice in which an individual trains their mind, or induces a different mode of consciousness, with the goal of either achieving a particular benefit, or clearing their mind from a lot of the 'clutter' that can prevent them from living their best life..

There are different forms of meditation. Some attempt to empty the mind of all conscious thought. Other forms encourage contemplation of a particular topic, such as the nature of human life. Still others encourage visualization.

Visualization/Guided Imagery

Visualization means to summon up a mental image, to see it in the 'mind's eye', as the common phrase goes. Research has shown numerous benefits to visualization, also referred to as guided imagery. Benefits include controlling pain, getting ready for athletic or other kinds of performances, relieving stress and anxiety, and more. Guided imagery can transform a negative mindset to a positive one, and therefore alter mood and perceptions.

Meditation and visualization are therefore two methods of training the mind to relieve stress and can be done separately or together.

Mindfulness

Mindfulness is a form of awareness in which you focus on the present moment. It can be used in meditation and visualization.

Most people live in the past, hung up on things that happened to them that they feel they can't move beyond. They also live in the future a lot of the time, making plans for their careers, families and so on, even though no person has any guarantee that they will even be alive tomorrow. As the saying goes, everyone dies with a to-do list.

Mindfulness enables you to slow down and live in the present for a short time. It also helps improve your focus so you can be present in each moment, such as when you are spending time with loved one. If you're washing the dishes, focus on the task as if it is the most important thing in the world. If you're spending time with loved ones, be mindful, and you will see that 30 minutes together can be more meaningful than hours in the same room not connecting with each other.

Deep Breathing

Deep breathing is one way to relax and slow down the body, or energize it. Short breaths when you are stressed make you ready for 'fight or flight'. Long, deep breaths help you become steadier and give you time to make a thoughtful decision rather than react on the spur of the moment.

It can be used on its own, or as a preliminary to meditation and/or visualization. Deep breathing is also part of yoga, which can be a great stress reliever.

Yoga

Yoga is a combination of meditation, visual imagery, deep breathing and physical movement and postures. It also teaches you to be mindful, such as of your body. All forms of exercise can relieve stress. Yoga uses your own body weight to tone and trim. It increases flexibility, lowers blood pressure, and promotes better sleep.

Tai chi

Tai chi is a martial art which is low impact and slow and meditative. It is great for improving the circulation, balance, strength and flexibility.

Quality Sleep

One final stress-relief technique is to aim for high-quality sleep. Every adult should have 8 to 9 hours of sleep per night. Quality sleep also means Rapid Eye Movement (REM) sleep, a deep form of sleep that helps you rest and rejuvenate more efficiently. Invest in a great mattress, pillows and everything to help you rest and recover each night.

A balanced diet, stress relief, exercise and a good night's sleep are all foundations of a healthy lifestyle and disease prevention. They can also help strengthen the digestive system and maintain the permeability of the gut.

One other important aspect is to maintain proper nutrition and regulate your eating habits. Treat your food as fuel. Crash diets, anorexia and bulimia can all have serious consequences, just like overeating.

CAM practitioners who have been investigating leaky gut have several suggestions for herbs and supplements that might be able to help with a leaky gut. Let's look a few of them in the next chapter.

Chapter 8 - Herbs and Supplements That Can Help

There are a number of herbs and supplements that have been suggested as able to help a leaky gut. Many of them focus on healing, and on firming up the gut in order to increase its impermeability. Suggestions include:

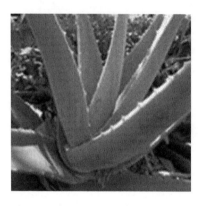

Aloe Vera

Aloe Vera is a healing plant often used to treat cuts, scrapes and burns. It is a spiny plant that can be grown almost anywhere, even in your home. When the spikes are cut, they exude a clear thick liquid/gel which can be applied to the skin. There are a number of drinks available on the market, but watch out for sugar. You can grow it yourself and add the gel to water or fruit juice in order to enhance internal health and healing. All health food stores and even Wal-Mart carries a good brand to use.

Butyrate

Butyrate comes from the Greek for butter, so it will give you an idea of the main source of this particular fatty acid that promotes healthy digestion in the small and especially the large intestine.

We all know fiber is supposed to be healthy for us, but it will work best in the right microbiome. You could consume more butter or goat cheese, but they will have an impact on your cholesterol levels. There are supplements, but they are expensive and poorly absorbed.

A better plan is to eat foods that encourage your body's own production of butyrate. These include:

Dark leafy greens
Vegetables

Insoluble fiber in grains such as:
Amaranth
Buckwheat
Millet
Oats
Quinoa

Low-fat dairy with active cultures can also help. Some experts also suggest coconut water and kefir. Fermented vegetables like kimchee (Korean pickled vegetables) and sauerkraut can also help.

These foods not only boost the microbiome, they decrease

inflammation, offering double the benefit for the same number of calories.

Collagen

Collagen is a building block for cell structures and maintains firmness, such as that of your skin. Therefore, CAM practitioners speculate that collagen could also help improve the impermeability of the intestines. Bone broth is an extremely popular way to get collagen in the food you eat. It's also easy to make and full of nutrition. Boil up and then simmer some bones, such as from a rotisserie chicken or turkey, with apple cider vinegar, for about 8 hours. Then drink as is or use in soups and stews.

Ginger

Ginger has been used in ancient medicine for thousands of years. It has warming and healing properties and has been associated with relief of arthritis and other inflammatory disorders. Use the fresh root or the dried and powdered form in a range of Indian and Chinese-style recipes.

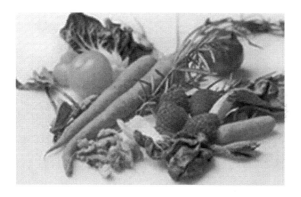

L-Glutamine

L-Glutamine is an important amino acid that the body uses in large amounts. It contributes to health in a number of ways, including:

•Improves gastrointestinal health because it is a vital nutrient that rebuilds and repairs

•Helps heal ulcers and leaky gut by boosting impermeability

•Serves as an essential neurotransmitter within the brain that helps with memory, focus and concentration, thus combating 'memory fog', which often accompanies autoimmune disorders and arthritic conditions such as fibromyalgia

•Improves IBS and diarrhea by balancing mucus production, which results in healthy bowel movements

•Promotes muscle growth and decreases muscle wastage, which happens as we age

•Helps maintain endurance during workouts

•Boosts metabolism

•Helps detoxify the body all the way down to the cellular level

•Improves athletic performance and recovery from endurance exercise

•Cuts cravings for sugar and for alcoholic beverages

•Improves blood sugar levels, important in relation to metabolic syndrome, pre-diabetes and diabetes

Natural sources include meat and poultry. Vegetable sources include:

- Beets
- Brussels sprouts
- Cabbage
- Carrots
- Kale
- Lentils, peas, beans and legumes
- Soybeans, tofu
- Spinach

Other main sources of L-glutamine include:

- Eggs, especially the whites
- Whole grains including oats, wheat germ and products made from whole wheat, quinoa, millet and brown rice.
- Nuts and nut butters, such as peanuts and peanut butter, almonds, pistachios, walnuts
- Seeds, such as pumpkin seeds and sunflower seeds

In most cases, people get more than enough L-glutamine via their ordinary diet. However, supplements are available and are recommended for people who have had surgery, especially gastrointestinal surgery. They are also given to people with extensive traumatic injuries and to cancer patients. High-endurance athletes will also use amino acid supplements that include L-glutamine.

If you are going to use a supplement, be sure to read the instructions and contraindications. Those with cirrhosis, liver disorders, epilepsy, and manic disorder should avoid it.

Licorice Root

Licorice root, which gives its flavor to black licorice, helps balance cortisol levels in the body and improves acid production in the stomach. It is also said to support the maintenance of the mucosal lining of the stomach. This herb is especially beneficial if someone's leaky gut is being caused by emotional stress. It is also used to treat diabetes.

However, it is important to note that licorice is a powerful herb which can have side effects even in small amounts. If you have heart health issues, high blood pressure, are on blood thinners, have kidney or liver issues, or are planning to have surgery, taking licorice can be risky.

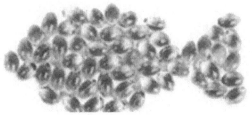

Omega-3s

As we discussed above, Omega-3s are anti-inflammatory and can soothe the gut. Oil also helps form an impermeable barrier, which can prevent leakage.

Omega-3s should not be taken if you have heart issues or are allergic to fish or shellfish. If you have the following health issues, you should avoid fish oil supplements:

- Bipolar disorder
- Depression
- Diabetes
- Heart issues

- High blood pressure
- HIV/AIDS
- Immune system disorders
- Liver disease

Prebiotics

See Chapter 6 above for more information.

Probiotics

See Chapter 6 above.

Quercetin

Quercetin is a plant pigment (flavonoid) which is found in many plants and foods, including:

- Apples
- Berries
- Buckwheat
- Green tea
- Gingko biloba

- St. John's Wort
- Onions
- Red wine

It is used for heart disease, diabetes, hay fever, peptic ulcer, inflammation, asthma, gout, viral infections, and chronic fatigue syndrome (CFS). Quercetin is also used to increase endurance and improve athletic performance. Large doses can cause kidney damage.

Turmeric

Turmeric is a bright yellow spice that has been used in Ayurvedic, (traditional Indian), medicine for about 5,000 years. Turmeric is tasty, and adds an interested flavor to Indian foods and rice dishes. It can be used in its fresh form, as a root, or dried and powdered.

Digestive enzymes

There are eight primary digestive enzymes, each designed to help break down different types of food:

1. Protease: Digests protein
2. Amylase: Digests carbohydrates
3. Lipase: Digests fats
4. Cellulase: Breaks down fiber
5. Maltase: Converts complex sugars from whole grains into glucose
6. Lactase: Digests milk sugar (lactose) in dairy products
7. Phytase: Helps with overall digestion, especially in extracting B vitamins
8. Sucrase: Digesting most sugars

Take your well-rounded digestive enzymes with food. Some people make a big deal of timing, but the bottom line is just to get them in around the time you're eating. Most people find it easiest to pop them just before they sit down to eat, but anytime within about

30 minutes of your meal is going to be beneficial, especially with large meals.

When you eat, your body has to break down the food into micro and macro nutrients that can then be absorbed and used by your body. Digestive enzymes are small proteins that act on specific molecules within foods to break them down. They really help your digestive tract in breaking down your food.

Your saliva is mainly made up of amylase. As the food passes through your system, protein is broken down by protease. Then the food passes to the small intestine, where the other enzymes do the rest. In a normally functioning small intestine, the nutrients from your food are absorbed into your bloodstream through millions of tiny villi in the wall of your gut. Think of them as the pile of a shag carpet.

However, in a leaky gut with low levels of enzymes, you will experience various symptoms, such as gas, bloating, acid reflux and more. Even if you do not have a leaky gut, your digestive enzyme production diminishes with age. This being the case, boosting your enzyme levels is a good idea and can also take the burden off your leaky gut.

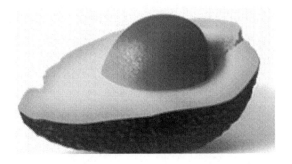

Enzyme-rich foods include:

- Avocado
- Bee pollen
- Coconut oil
- Dairy products with live cultures
- Extra virgin olive oil
- Grapes
- Kiwi
- Mango
- Papaya
- Pineapple

If you've ever tried to make a Jell-O salad with kiwi or pineapple, you will know it doesn't work. This is because the high level of enzymes break down or basically start to digest the gelatin before it ever sets, so you can see how powerful these foods can be.

Other suggestions for boosting your enzymes are to:

- Eat a range of raw fruits and vegetables
- Don't overeat
- Chew slowly and thoroughly
- Avoid chewing gum, which stimulates enzyme production because it thinks the body is getting food, but then they go to waste

Organic Salts

Organic salts, or tissue salts, are vital minerals that perform many functions in the body. They are commonly referred to as electrolytes and need to be replenished regularly for the body to perform all of its essential functions.

Organic salts include calcium, sodium, potassium, magnesium and phosphorous, on their own and in various combinations with one another. Phosphorous helps repair cells and tissues and could be very beneficial for leaky gut syndrome. A homeopath can help you with organic salts, but always try to get them through the food you eat first, rather than through supplementation.

If your stomach is very acidic, try:

- Apples
- Apricots
- Asparagus
- Carrots
- Grapes
- Peaches
- Raspberries
- Strawberries

If you often get cramps or heartburn, try:

- Bananas
- Figs
- Green leafy vegetables
- Lentils
- Oranges
- Walnuts

If you tend to have a nervous stomach, try eating more:

- Apples
- Broccoli
- Cauliflower
- Dates
- Garlic
- Guavas
- Lemons
- Oats
- Olives
- Onions

Hydrochloric Acid Supplements

The stomach produces hydrochloric acid that helps to digest your food and also kill many potentially harmful bugs that could be in it. However, if acid levels aren't strong enough, it will be harder for the food to break down, leading to poor absorption of nutrients. It can also mean delayed emptying of the stomach, which can lead to a range of uncomfortable digestive symptoms. A side note: Approximately 30% of your energy is used every day to digest your food. Take care of your stomach and your stomach will take care of you.

If you think you might have a low level of hydrochloric acid, avoid drinking liquids with your meals. If that still doesn't work, try a supplement. Apple cider vinegar is commonly used to help lose weight but it can also aid digestion and relieve arthritis symptoms. We use and recommend Bragg's Organic Raw Apple

Cider Vinegar. It's aids in digestion and is rich in enzymes and potassium. It can be purchased almost everywhere now. Here's an Amazon link for you too. Amazon-Braggs

If you still don't seem to have enough stomach acid, there are a number of supplements available on the market that you can take with each meal. Finding the optimal dose can take some time and experimentation. You can take it one pill at a time until you get to the point where you start to feel like you have heartburn. In this case, take one less pill and track how you feel in your food diary.

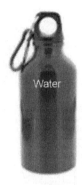

Pure water

We should try drink 1 ounce of pure water for every two pounds of body weight example 128 pounds, then you would drink 64 ounces of water each day, just for maintenance since our bodies are 60-65% water. If your weight is 200 pounds then 100 ounces of water for maintenance is needed or 12 eight-ounce glasses of fresh water every day. The trouble with this is that not all water is created equal. Tap water has a variety of minerals in it depending on where you live. Some water is 'hard' with a great deal of minerality, while other water is termed soft.

In addition, tap water is often treated with chlorine and fluoride, the former to prevent bacteria in the water, and the latter added to improve dental health. Both of these minerals have been suggested as possible causes of leaky gut, malabsorption of nutrients, and damage to the metabolism. Scientists who compared countries which did not fluoridate the water with those which did had far fewer obese people and ones suffering from digestive disorders.

Plus, if you have a leaky gut, drinking a lot of liquid will only increase the chance of leakage. Having said that, water is your best beverage of choice compared to soda, fruit juice, or other sugary drinks, and is definitely better for you than energy drinks and alcohol. (Health Note: if this year you make one small choice to improve your health, focus on soda pop. They are empty calories with no-upside for your body's health. When you quit soda pop, you will likely lose weight and begin to feel better immediately after the caffeine withdrawal phase.)

The trouble with bottled water is that some of it can be even less pure than what's already coming out of your tap, plus you have to lug it back and forth from the market. Invest in a filter like Pur® or Zero® Water filters that you put on your tap, or a couple of filtering jugs. Change the filters regularly according to the instructions. When used correctly, the filters can remove nearly 100% of the impurities in the water.

Another effective way to get the hydration your body needs that has a positive effect of leaky gut symptoms is the use of alkaline water. You may have heard some of the various health claims about alkaline water. Some say it can help slow the aging process, regulate your body's pH level, and prevent chronic diseases like cancer. But what exactly is alkaline water, and why all the hype?

The "alkaline" in alkaline water refers to its pH level. The pH level is a number that measures how acidic or alkaline a substance is on a scale of 0 to 14. For example, something with a pH of 1 would be very acidic, and something with a pH of 14 would be very alkaline. Most people's pH is around 7.0. (You can test your pH easily with a saliva pH test strip that can be purchased anywhere).

Alkaline water has a higher pH level than regular drinking water. Because of this, some advocates of alkaline water believe it can neutralize the acid in your body. Normal drinking water generally has a neutral pH of around 7. Alkaline water typically has a pH of 8 or 9.5. There are alkaline water machines from $1000-

$6000 that can produce a number of different water pH values, and then there are vendors that are selling the alkaline water in bottles in most health food and upscale grocery stores.

Despite the lack of proven scientific research, proponents of drinking alkaline water still believe in its many proposed health benefits, which include:

- anti-aging properties (via liquid antioxidants that absorb more quickly into the human body)
- colon-cleansing properties
- immune system support
- hydration, skin health, and other detoxifying properties
- weight loss
- cancer resistance

Save large 2-liter or gallon containers and keep a supply of filtered water ready any time you need it. Consider buying a stainless steel water bottle for each member of the family so they can always have filtered water with them. Drink a little throughout the day to stay hydrated. Don't drink too much as one time, especially before or during a meal.

For people trying to lose weight who fill up on water to try to feel full so they will eat less, do it 2 hours after a meal so you don't interfere with your digestion.

Drinking before bedtime can be problematic because you may have to wake up several times in the middle of the night to urinate, so judge your consumption accordingly. If you have to urinate often at night, consider avoiding liquids after 9pm.

Water is an essential part of blood, filtration of the blood to remove toxins, and the digestive process, but impurities could be contribution to your leaky gut. Start drinking more water which you have filtered and note any changes in your symptoms in your food journal.

Conclusion

Leaky gut has only recently been recognized by mainstream doctors, in the same way that they ignored Lyme disease and fibromyalgia for decades until there was enough medical evidence to demonstrate that these symptoms were not all in their patient's minds, but were actually a sign of a genuine medical condition.

In the case of leaky gut, we can't be certain if it is a condition of its own, or associated with other medical conditions. But one thing is for sure. We don't want to sit around being ill and miserable until medical professionals finally start paying attention to us and taking our complaints seriously.

CAM practitioners such as homeopaths, functional medicine doctors, naturopaths, Ayurvedic and traditional Chinese medicine practitioners work with people suffering from leaky gut and offer them safe, effective relief through food, drink, herbs and supplements, as well as lifestyle measures.

If you've been struggling with a range of digestive issues and unexplained symptoms, start and keep a food journal. These are very inexpensive and there are many choices on places like Amazon to begin. Then review what you've learned in this book and start putting it into practice. Write down the foods you've added to your menus, and the ones you've removed. Try an anti-inflammatory diet and healing foods. Then see what a difference they make to your health.

Please also know, that "YOU are the best doctor of YOU!" There is no one alive that knows you and your health better than you do, including your spouse. Have confidence in knowing how you feel by letting those that care for your health know too. You are unique and wonderful. It's noteworthy to know that not everyone responds to the same treatments, drugs, supplements or protocols. Because of that, do your own research confidently. Ask questions of your medical professionals. If they know, they'll tell you. You'll find in many cases, that your research will be cutting edge and that your medical professional may not even be aware of how to help you naturally. That's okay. Our medical professionals are very busy these days and can't keep up with everything in the medical world.

Also, please consider natural alternatives first in your evaluation process, before opting for a "quick medical solution." In some cases, the medical option may be the only choice that makes sense for you. So, consider that. We certainly have found that 21st century natural approaches to our health works in most cases and certainly in the case of leaky gut works best. Medical pharmaceutical treatments and surgeries have their place, but in the case of surgeries, there's no going back to a natural protocol after a surgery. Perhaps, adopt the philosophy in your life, as we have, when we say, "go natural first". You'll probably be better off for it in the long run, and you'll always be able to consider a medical approach later on if you choose.

I hope this makes sense to you. Overall, from our experiences, natural approaches are generally less expensive and in many cases less invasive too. You only have "one body" so it's imperative to care for it the very best you can.

As we come to the end of this book, we want to thank you for your decision to learn more about this leaky gut condition and heal it. This condition is real. And it affects so many people, worldwide. With your new understanding, please reach out and help others who are also suffering with leaky gut.

To your best self in life and in health!

Bob

P.S. One final request. Please leave a positive comment and a 5-Star review, if you would. It would truly help us to reach new patients and keep us writing new books on conditions that affect our lives so completely. Thank you!

Resources

Leaky Gut Syndrome
http://www.webmd.com/digestive-disorders/features/leaky-gut-syndrome

Leaky Gut Syndrome
http://www.nhs.uk/conditions/leaky-gut-syndrome/Pages/Introduction.aspx

Fish Oil Side Effects and Interactions
http://wb.md/2cc0jGm

L-Glutamine
http://wb.md/28WyDFE

Butyrate
http://bodyecology.com/articles/add-these-fiber-rich-foods-to-your-diet-to-fight-inflammation

Licorice Root
http://wb.md/2mNzAUt

https://blog.kettleandfire.com/ Kettle and Fire has a very nice blog with tips on meal planning, bone broth soups etc. Check them out.

https://www.ncbi.nlm.nih.gov/pmc/articles/PMC5440529/ Many citations and research studies on the leaky gut and autoimmune connection. Well researched.

http://www.mercola.com/ Dr. Joseph Mercola is a master health care practitioner that is committed to providing the most up-to-date natural health information and resources that will most benefit you. You'll love his work.

https://draxe.com/ Dr. Josh Axe has taken the health world by storm. Must read site for great recipes, health news, functional fitness and many health topics.

FINAL THOUGHTS

Thank you so much for taking time out to learn more about Leaky Gut Syndrome and your health.

It's a serious and often, overlooked condition that can completely take over and change your life. If we can get a handle on it, by RECOGNIZING the symptoms, REMOVING the foods and factors that damage the gut (triggers), REPLACE the damaging foods with healing foods, REPAIR your leaky gut with specific herbs and supplements and REBALANCE your gut flora with prebiotics and probiotics and helpful enzymes, and are consistent and mindful in your approach towards your leaky gut condition, you'll begin to experience improvement very quickly.

Remember, you're the best doctor of you! No one knows your health situation as well as you. Trust your "gut" (pun intended) but continue to consult those who have knowledge in such things. General Practioners today are really overwhelmed with their patient flow. New ideas and protocols in health are being developed daily. Physicians, or anyone for that matter, find it hard to keep up on every detail in their own medical fields, let alone alternative medical protocols and treatments. Be a good student too. Continue to learn what you can about your health and your body and then set in motion a plan to achieve your health goals.

Share your goals with your family, friends and healthcare professionals so that they can help you achieve them. Find accountability partners too, that will go with you to the gym regularly, who will keep you on your diet path, who will be there when you need to call someone to talk to.

Please also consider investing a couple of dollars, at the beginning of your journey, in a health journal. A food/health journal will:

- Help you notice patterns
- Notice foods that aggravate your system
- You can't change what you can't measure
- Keep you from backsliding into a rut
- Easier to stay on track
- See how lifestyle factors affect food intake and vice versa
- Have an objective record you can look back on later.

I'll have my food/health journal out soon, for you so please check back. It'll be the best of the best and affordable.

Let me leave with a ten quotes that I love that may relate to your health.

- Your health is your wealth
- If you don't take care of your body, where are you going to live?
- Let food be thy medicine, and medicine be thy food. ~Hippocrates
- Just because you're not sick, doesn't mean you're healthy.
- Those who think they have no time for exercise, will sooner or later have to find time for illness. ~Edward Stanley
- From the bitterness of disease man learns the sweetness of health.
- The doctor of the future will no longer treat the human frame with drugs, but rather will cure and prevent disease with nutrition. ~Thomas Edison

- A man too busy to take care of his health, is like the mechanic that's too busy to take care of his tools.
- True healthcare reform starts in the kitchen, not in Washington D.C.
- I believe that the greatest gift you can give your family and the world is a healthy you. ~Joyce Meyer

Once again thank you for beginning your journey with us here. Please leave a positive comment on Amazon, if you have found this helpful.

To your best health ever...

Bob Armstrong

Notes:

Notes:

Manufactured by Amazon.ca
Bolton, ON